UBIQUITOUS

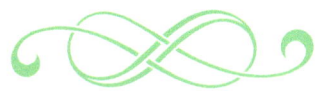

Apple Juice, Lemon Juice, Olive Oil

Sharon R. Leippi

Balboa Press books may be ordered through booksellers or by contacting:

Balboa Press
A Division of Hay House
1663 Liberty Drive
Bloomington, IN 47403
www.balboapress.com
1 (877) 407-4847

ISBN: 978-1-5043-9594-6 (sc)
ISBN: 978-1-5043-9595-3 (e)

Print information available on the last page.

Balboa Press rev. date: 01/23/2018

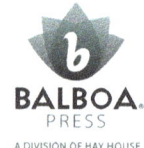

BALBOA
PRESS
A DIVISION OF HAY HOUSE

Edited by Attorney John C. Pharr

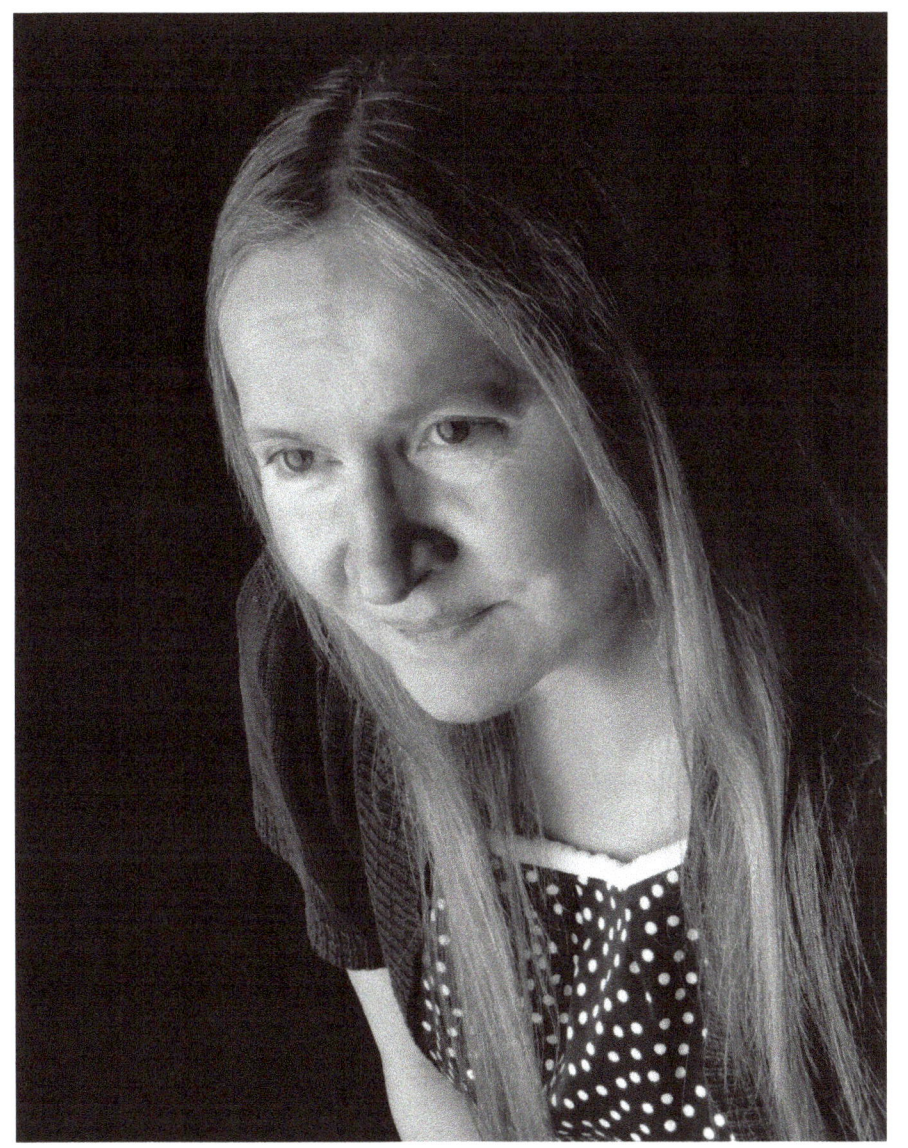

Introduction

Apple Juice, Lemon Juice, Olive Oil.

These three ingredients saved my life.

How? I don't really know.

This simple, natural home remedy is ubiquitous – widespread throughout the world; available from some health professionals; found over the Internet – even on Quackwatch.

I am not the only one who has experienced positive results from apple juice, lemon juice, and olive oil. I personally know several people who have greatly benefited. But I've also met many people who have never even heard of this simple, natural home remedy.

That's the reason I'm writing this book.

I haven't encountered anyone complaining of any adverse side effects from the process in Chapter 5 – but, please, consult your family physician before going forward with it – because I don't want to be sued; thanx.

1
Feeling Bad !

The year was 2011. The place was Anchorage, Alaska. I was working for two attorneys and in 2011, all three of us had been ill. Attorney John C. Pharr ended up in hospital on heavy duty antibiotics after contracting MRSA (most likely from working out at a health club – against doctors' advice) following foot surgery. Attorney Lance C. Wells landed in the ICU for a week with a diagnosis of septic shock, following pneumonia and overdoing it, and a prognosis of 50/50 recovery. And I was declining day by day with more and more symptoms – to the point that I thought I was dying. I was 54 years old.

2

My Symptoms

I was sick for a year. I was puzzled that I had such strange symptoms, but why? I had ordered a (harmless) colon cleanse product off the TV – perhaps this was the instigator. After taking the product, throughout the year I experienced the following symptoms:

- Abdominal discomfort and a feeling of fullness;
- Fatigue;
- Mucous in throat;
- Burping;
- Constipation and foul smelling gas;
- Cold hands – so I would wear gloves indoors;
- Waiting over an hour every morning to open up my hands;
- Painful thumb when writing;
- Pain on walking – I actually printed out an application for handicapped parking permit;
- Severe acid reflux to the point I bought over-the-counter (OTC) medication;
- Twenty-pound weight gain;
- Feeling of impending doom;
- Finally I could not bend over.

Getting Checked Out

At one point in the summer, I had called my family physician's office to set an appointment to see my doctor, who was an internist.

During the physical exam, she wanted to check "the gallbladder" and so she palpated the right upper quadrant of my abdomen but could not detect anything out of the ordinary. There was no pain on palpation. Vital signs – normal. I left the doctor's office and went home. Blood work – normal.

4

Burgers and French Fries

A delivery of burgers and French fries to the law offices where I worked was a pivotal moment. I ate some French fries. Later that day I felt abdominal discomfort.

I realized that French fries are considered "high fat" – could this be a trigger for a gallbladder symptom?

I called my friend, Sharon from Minnesota, who had experienced positive results from an apple juice, lemon juice, olive oil natural home remedy provided by her chiropractor. She told me what she had used. I also checked out the Internet and read testimonials from people, even from Europe, who gave instructions for an apple juice, lemon juice, olive oil home remedy. I remembered how Marlene, a friend from Canada, described decades ago how she "remedied a gallbladder problem" with apple juice, lemon juice, and olive oil.

I analyzed it all and gave myself the green light to try for the first time this ubiquitous remedy.

I never did find out who sent the burgers and French fries. Would the sender of the burgers and French fries please contact the offices so you can be properly thanked.

Taking Action

Day 1:

I drank apple juice and ate apples, especially granny smith apples.

I ate about a dozen prunes and drank a cup of senna leaf tea.

I didn't eat or drink anything else.

Day 2:

I drank apple juice and ate apples, especially granny smith apples.

Day 3:

I drank apple juice and ate apples, especially granny smith apples.

At the end of Day 3, I combined in blender one-half cup fresh lemon juice and one-half cup EVOO (olive oil) at room temperature and drank it.

After brushing my teeth, I lay on my right side with knees to my chest for several hours and then for most of the night.

Day 4:

In the morning, I ate a few prunes and drank a cup of senna leaf tea.

I resumed eating and drinking and had breakfast.

6

Feeling Good !

I got my life back after taking the apple juice, lemon juice, olive oil natural home remedy (beginning of November). I felt fine again. Over the Christmas holidays, I repeated the process for peace of mind, just to ensure that I did all I could. I remained symptom-free but six months later I went through the process again, for peace of mind and as a preventative.

I had no adverse reaction from this simple, natural home remedy. There were no side effects. I personally chose not to include Epsom salts because I felt the ingredient may be too harsh.

I am so relieved that I don't have to wait an hour every morning to open up my hands. I can walk and write without pain. I can bend over. No more acid reflux. My weight is back to normal.

I still have my gallbladder. I didn't need emergency gallbladder surgery.

This happened seven years ago. All symptoms completely vanished after taking apple juice, lemon juice, and olive oil. I've never felt better in my life. I am now 61.

More Simple, Natural Home Remedies

- Vitamin E applied topically to a cat scratch *worked for me* to help prevent scarring.
- Daily use of unwaxed dental floss and narrow toothbrush *worked for me* to help heal bleeding gums.
- A small amount of minced fresh garlic, taken on a spoon and swallowed with water or fruit juice, *worked for me* to help stop a coughing spell.
- Aloe vera gel (gel inside the aloe vera plant leaf, or bottled gel) *worked for me* to help soothe sunburn.
- An apple cider vinegar rinse before shampooing (apple cider vinegar diluted with water) *worked for me* to help remedy dandruff.
- A cup of senna leaf tea *worked for me* to help remedy constipation.
- A cup of green tea *worked for me* to help quench thirst and doubled as a health promoter.
- Starting the day with a mug of fresh lemon juice, honey, and distilled or spring water (heated or at room temperature) *worked for me* to help break the fast from the night before.

Medical Disclaimer

This book is not intended to provide medical advice or diagnose, cure, mitigate, treat, or prevent any disease. *Ubiquitous: Apple Juice, Lemon Juice, Olive Oil* does not replace your physician, psychiatrist, and pharmacist.

About the Author

Sharon Leippi has always been interested in natural home remedies. Having a registered nurse background and an Associate of Science degree from Southern Adventist University, Collegedale, Tennessee (alum '82), her interest in health promotion continues with this book.

Sharon is the author of Fire & Ice: ALASKA – Baked, Blended, & Sautéed (Frosty Books) where the apple juice, lemon juice, olive oil natural home remedy is featured on page 138 of her cookbook.

She has written Think Hope Live: Embracing Life – Defeating Suicide, and also Road Tripping from Alaska to New York City: Journaling the Journey & Taking Pix Along the Way. (Balboa Press).

www.ingramcontent.com/pod-product-compliance
Lightning Source LLC
Chambersburg PA
CBHW041132280526
45792CB00013B/2400